Homemade Hand Sanitizer

How Make Homemade Hand Sanitizer

ELISABETH STOONES

recipient reader. Under no circumstances will any legal responsibility or blame be held against the publisher for any reparation, damages, or monetary loss due to the information herein, either directly or indirectly.

Respective authors own all copyrights not held by the publisher.

The information herein is offered for informational purposes solely, and is universal as so. The presentation of the information is without contract or any type of guarantee assurance.

The trademarks that are used are without any consent, and the publication of the trademark is without permission or backing by the trademark owner. All trademarks and brands within this book are for clarifying purposes only and are the owned by the owners themselves, not affiliated with this document

Table of Contents

CHAPTER ONE

Sanitation and Hygiene

Sanitation and hygiene are essential to health, survival, and development. Numerous countries are a little bit incapable of providing satisfactory sanitation to their whole populations, leaving people in danger for water, sanitation, and hygiene (WASH)- related diseases and infections. All through the world, an expected 2.4 billion people need essential sanitation (over 32% of the total populace). Basic hygiene is depicted as approaching offices for the removal of human waste (feces and urine), as well as being able to keep up with hygienic conditions everywhere, through services like garbage removal, industrial/hazardous waste management, and water treatment.

Sanitation has to do with general health conditions identified with clean drinking water and adequate treatment and removal of human excreta and sewage. Preventing human contact with contaminated sources is a type of sanitation, as is handwashing with soap. Sanitation frameworks intend to secure human health and well-being by coming up with a solution or cure that will stop the transmission of disease, mainly through the fecal-oral route. For instance, diarrhea, a very important reason for ailing health and hindered development in kids, can be decreased through sanitation. Numerous different diseases can be transmitted in communities that have low levels of sanitation and hygiene, for instance, ascariasis (a kind of intestinal worm disease), cholera, hepatitis, polio, and trachoma, to say but a few.

Home Hygiene; Tips, Tricks, and Best Practices

Know how germs are spread. Knowing how diseases are spread from one individual to the next is the initial phase in proper home hygiene to forestall the spread of sickness. This fact sheet from the Centers for disease control and prevention offers helpful data on how germs (and in this manner, disease) are spread from one person to the other– principally through small drops made when people talk, sniffle, or cough. Hygiene is essential to forestall the spread of germs, sickness, and infections, even with the use of vaccines and antibiotics. While present-day medication goes far in preventing and treating disease, this book also calls attention to that families share a significant obligation in avoidance.

A 2008 meta-analysis found that an increase in personal and home hygiene brings about a 31% decrease in gastrointestinal disease and a 21% decrease in respiratory illnesses. High-traffic areas of our home and items that are touched often are germ banks. As per WebMD, one investigation found that the kitchen sink has a higher number of microorganisms than the toilet or trash can.

Tips for Properly Cleaning the Surfaces in Your Home and Prevent the Spread of Illness

The accompanying resources offer helpful information on how to appropriately clean the surfaces and items in your home to forestall the spread of germs and sicknesses.

- Clean and purify the much of the time contacted surfaces in your home routinely when somebody is debilitated. You should typically clean your home in any case, yet, it's especially critical to ensure the surfaces relatives' touch regularly are disinfected when a relative is sick.

- Cleaning removes dirt and grime, purifying, and eliminating germs. As this book clarifies, a few items ought to be cleaned to expel dirt and then disinfected, which removes a few germs. Surfaces in bathrooms, toys, dishes, and silverware ought to be both cleaned and purified.

- Hygienic cleaning practices help to forestall the spread of germs and diseases. Hygienic cleaning includes centering your endeavors in the territories where germs are well on the way to spread from and cause contamination. It's additionally essential to perceive that great home hygiene isn't a once-week by week, profound cleaning, however, a continuous piece of your day by day life.

- If kids fall sick, give them hard-surface toys that are anything but difficult to clean. Urging kids to play with simple to-clean toys when they're sick means it's simpler for you to downplay the spread of germs.

- Cleaning "as-you-go" permits you to remove dirt in high-hazard regions. "Cleaning is significant as germs don't have any place to live once dirt has been evacuated. You should clean routinely (especially in high-hazard zones), every day rather than once in a week. You have to clean areas like the kitchen and washroom 'as you go.' You don't have to scrub floors as frequently as you clean high-hazard zones.

- Clean down surfaces like countertops in your home every day with cleaning solutions or sterilizing wipes. This book offers a variety of helpful hints for keeping your home spotless and clean when a relative or guest is debilitated, including room-by-room cleaning tips. For example, you should utilize paper towels for drying your hands after washing, or at the very least, use a different towel for each member of the family– and wash them weekly.

- Microwave your sponges is important. Microwave your sponges on high for 2 minutes each week will help clean them, or you can settle on a five-minute soak in a bleach solution. The microwave strategy has even been shown to kill 99% of bacteria. Few of the most germ-friendly spots in your home, including those you don't consider as often as possible, for example, cutting boards, bathmats, and the coffee maker.

- Try not to disregard the windows and doorway tracks. These regions tend to accommodate residues, dirt, and dead bugs, and not keeping them clean can make you increasingly vulnerable to colds and respiratory ailments.

Picking the Right Cleaning Products and Proper Handling

The following resources give data on choosing the best cleaning items, how to utilize cleaning items fittingly for most extreme viability and dealing with tips to guarantee your health when using cleaning items and chemical solutions around the home. The flu is exceptionally frail outside the body when presented to air, however sterilizing very well surfaces (where the virus can survive, for example, doorknobs, countertops, consoles, remote controls, toys, and similar items is a smart thought.

Bleach is a very cheap and effective disinfecting agent. Bleach can kill some of the dangerous and highly hazardous bacteria, for example, staphylococcus, streptococcus, E. coli, and salmonella. Search for surface-disinfecting sprays that are EPA-registered for eliminating germs on hard surfaces. Items that kills the Influenza A virus will also be successful against the H1N1 flu strain.

Vinegar hasn't been tried as widely as chlorine bleach, yet it is a sanitizing choice for people who favor natural items. As indicated by Rodale's Organic Life, "The vinegar you purchase in stores, regardless of whether it is apple cider, balsamic, white, or any other type, contains 5% acidic content, which has antimicrobial properties." Some investigations have demonstrated that vinegar, utilized in blend with table salt or hydrogen peroxide, can restrain the development of certain strains of E. coli, and it's likewise a compelling mold killer. In the case of choosing vinegar, white distilled vinegar is your most logical option. ToxinAlert.com calls attention to the fact that as a result of its acidity levels, white distilled vinegar is successful at killing bacteria, mold, and germs, and it's also environmentally friendly.

In the wake of recuperating from sickness, it's critical to clean the overlooked regions. Wash pillows and bedding in high temp water, replace or clean your toothbrush, and wipe down the refrigerator handle, to say but a few.

Disinfecting wipes are convenient to keep around the house, especially for tricks like cleaning down your credit and debit cards. Toys and similar objects small items with hard surfaces can be sanitized by soaking them from a detergent and water solution. Blend one tablespoon of bleach in with one gallon of water for the ideal purifying solution for toys.

Individual Hygiene and Self-Care Tips to Prevent Illness

HOMEMADE HAND SANITIZER

The following resources provide informations on personal hygiene tips to follow to abstain from spreading germs and diseases to others, especially when more than two people cohabitate in the same room or apartment.

- Maintain distance from contact with others; however much as could be expected when you're sick, particularly if you have a sickness that can be deadly. It's anything but difficult to maintain a strategic distance from contact with individuals grinding away or school by remaining at home, yet your other relatives will have a similar space. Staying in a room or one part of the home will lessen the germs spread all through the house.

- Cover your mouth when you cough. Something as basic as covering your mouth and nose with a tissue when you cough or sniffle can assist with forestalling the spread of germs to people around you.

- Utilize legitimate hand-washing methods. Mostly washing your hand isn't sufficient to dispose of illness-causing germs and microorganisms. This book from the Centers for Disease Control and Prevention traces appropriate hand-washing systems.

- That implies washing your hands for at least 20 seconds with cleanser and water. As this article calls attention to, one examination saw the standard hand-washing time as only six seconds. It's likewise imperative to make sure to clean between your fingers and under your fingernails.

- Liquor based hand sanitizers are a successful method to keep up hand sanitation without cleanser and water. Alcohol-based hand sanitizers "fundamentally diminish the number of pathogens on the skin.

Appropriate Nutrition and Food Handling Tips to Beat Illness and Stay Healthy

Diet and food are essential when you're sick just as when somebody in your family is sick. The following resources offer supporting data on the best nutrition and food handling practices to help you and your family remain healthy.

- Clean your hands with soap before touching or eating food. Individuals regularly become sick by getting germs from basic surfaces and afterward contacting their mouth, nose, or eyes. So whether you're ill or somebody in your family is, washing your hands before touching or eating food can assist you with abstaining from spreading ailment or becoming ill.

- If you have food poisoning, you ought to abstain from touching or preparing food until 48 hours after you have recuperated. On the off chance that touching and preparing food is unavoidable, follow the tips laid out here including, washing your hands with soap and water and drying them with a different towel before making food.

- Separate raw meats from other foods. "Cross-contamination can happen when microorganisms are spread, starting with one food item then onto the next. This is particularly usual when taking care of raw meat, poultry,eggs and fish. The important is to keep these foods—and their juices—away from ready-to-eat food sources," as indicated by the FDA.

- Norovirus is the primary source of ailment and outbreaks from contaminated foods in the United States. As indicated by the CDC, food can become contaminated when affected individuals who have vomit on their hands touch the food, when food is set on countertops or different surfaces that have an infectious stool or vomit on them, or when tiny drops of vomit from a contaminated individual splash through the air and land on food. These methods of contamination points to the significance of legitimate hygiene for both individuals and family surfaces.

- Follow great defrosting, stockpiling, and cooking practices for transient foods, specifically. Cooking meals at the wrong temperature or not refrigerating perishable foods within two hours (or one hour if the temperature is over 90 degrees fahrenheit) are only two of the numerous tips offered by the U.S. Division of Agriculture. Read more to get more information on defrosting systems, and on neatness and food handling best practices.

- Wash vegetables and natural products before eating them. This is particularly significant for products of the soil that won't be cooked. "Abstain from eating alfalfa sprouts until their security can be guaranteed. Strategies to disinfect alfalfa seeds and sprouts are being explored," prescribes WebMD.

- Utilize a thermometer to ensure meat and poultry (including ground meat and poultry) are cooked in the best possible temperatures. Fish ought to be prepared until it is soft and flaky when eaten with a fork.

- By seeing how germs spread and cause sickness and finding a way to keep your home clean, forestalling colds, diseases, and viruses from spreading through your entire family is no longer an impossible feat. Being determined about keeping up a spotless, healthy home is as simple as keeping steady over keeping common areas and frequently touched surfaces very clean and using a touch of additional caution when somebody in your home falls sick.

Personal Hygiene

Getting and keeping clear skin is very simpler than you might suspect. Get these sound propensities to help expel breakouts.

1. Wash your face two times every day.

Both over-washing and under-washing can mean something bad for your skin. The ideal amount of time one should wash it is twice.

2. Eat a reasonable and sound diet.

You eat to keep up a solid weight yet eating the correct nourishment can likewise support your skin. Eating certain nourishments and beverages may make skin break out. Scientists are exploring in the case of eating certain sugars, for example,white potatoes, potatoes,chips, cornflakes, pretzels, and drinking skim milk may exacerbate skin break out.

3. Make sure to clean up after a workout.

Exercise is acceptable for your body as well as for your skin, as well, since it can improve dissemination. Simply remember to shower and wash your face after a decent workout, so microscopic organisms, and dead skin cells don't obstruct your pores.

4. Use an oil-free moisturizer.

Moisturizers help keep your skin from drying out, which can make more oil be delivered. Search for lightweight, without oil items that won't stop up pores.

5. Don't forget the sunscreen.

The sun's UV rays dry out your skin, so your body responds by delivering more oil. Also, you realize what more oil implies. All the more critically, presentation to the sun's UV rays can cause skin malignant growth. So do yourself tremendous support and never go out without sunscreen. Just make sure it's oil-free!

Face and Body Hygiene

It ought to likewise be noticed that;

- More than half of sound individuals have Staphylococcus aureus living in or on their nasal sections, throats, hair, or skin.

- Within the underlying 15 minutes of washing, the normal individual sheds 6 x 106 Colony Forming Units (CFU) of Staphylococcus aureus.

- The ordinary individual swimmer contributes at any rate of 0.14 grams of fecal material to the water, generally, inside the initial 15 minutes of entering. Have a Shower with soap before swimming helps stop the spread of germs by expelling fecal material from the body.

- Trachoma, the essential wellspring of preventable visual weakness around the globe, is related to the nonattendance of facial hygiene.

- Inadequate contact lens hygiene, for instance, failure to properly purify contact lens, is related to an expanded danger of acquiring the eye disease Acanthamoeba keratitis.

- The spread of pinworms can be diminished by legitimate hygiene, including cutting nails and showering kids quickly they get up in the first part of the day.

- Hundreds of thousands of individuals in the U.K. (someplace in the scope of 1.2% and 1.3% of the all-out populace) secure external ear illnesses consistently, on account of contaminated water remaining in the ear in the wake of swimming or washing.

CHAPTER TWO

Healthy habits

Top Ten Daily Habits

Numerous individuals spend a fortune on beautifying agents and skincare items wanting to accomplish a decent complexion. What they neglect to acknowledge, in any case, is that healthy and excellent skin starts with a proper skincare routine. An examination of the evolving job of skincare uncovered this reality. In the study, it was discovered that one's daily skincare routine positively affects the general nature of an individual's complexion, particularly if it is the case that it is bolstered by effective products. To help you on your mission for a delightful and radiant complexion, here are 10 daily skincare habits that you should practice for healthy, radiant skin:

1. DRINK PLENTY OF WATER

Drinking plenty of water isn't just the most fundamental skincare habit, it is also an essential habit for keeping up general physical health too. The cells in our body are generally comprised of water, and water plays a fundamental job in keeping up the physiological balance. Considering these realities alone, scientists have investigated the relationship between water and healthy complexion. Drinking water won't just satisfy your thirst, but it will keep your skin appropriately hydrated too. One ongoing examination distributed in the Journal of Clinical, Cosmetic, and Investigational Dermatology supports the skin-hydrating impacts of drinking a lot of water.

In the clinical study, 49 healthy ladies were grouped in two. The subjects in a single gathering were made to drink at least 5.2 liters of water a day while the other group just drank under 3.2 liters of water daily. After watching and testing the subject's skin hydration for a month, the scientists reasoned that consuming a high volume of water every day exponentially increases the hydration level of the skin. Completely hydrated skin is clear with barely visible pores, practically no defects, and radiant to the eye. So as opposed to drinking coffee, juice, or other packaged beverages, it's ideal to drink water. Aside from its skin benefits, water is free from calories and drinking a greater amount of it can assist you with skipping drinks that are filled with calories, hence helping you keep up a healthy weight.

2. APPLY SUNSCREEN

Sunscreen is any substance or item that shields your skin from the damaging effects of the sun's ultraviolet rays. While the sun's rays can cause you to feel more energetic and alluring when you get a tan, you ought to abstain from going out without wearing sunscreen. Exposure to the sun's ultraviolet rays negatively impacts the state of your skin. Indeed, the vast majority of the signs that are related to skin aging are more often the effects of increased exposure to sunlight. UV rays damage the skin's flexible and collagen tissue, which brings about skin sagging, stretching, and wrinkles. It additionally causes spots, skin staining, age spots, and even skin disease. Try to imagine what your skin must be experiencing when you go out under the sun without proper sunscreen protection.

For a long time, sunscreen has been known principally for viably shielding the skin from developing any indications of skin maturing. An ongoing report uncovered that the continual use of sunscreen even gives advantageous consequences on the photo-aged skin (or damaged skin because of sun presentation). Specialists found that subjects who ceaselessly wear sunscreen for 18 months encounter very rapid improvement in their skin condition. It should be noted that sunscreen possibly works only if it is the case that you pick the correct one and if you apply it accurately. The American Academy of Dermatology (AAD) prescribes a sunscreen item with SPF of 30 or higher, water-safe, and gives protection against both UVA and UVB rays. Make a point to apply a liberal amount of sunscreen to all exposed skin 15 minutes before you go out and try to reapply at regular intervals to help your skin remain protected.

3. PRACTICE GOOD EATING HABITS

Your skin condition is an extension of what is happening inside your body, which means to have a ravishing and radiant complexion; you ought to appropriately nourish your body. This reality had, for quite some time, been built up the same number of food specialists have demonstrated the positive association between good food and youthful-looking skin. Given this reality, you ought to incorporate eating skin-friendly foods into your skincare routine. Such foods include vegetables and fruits that are plentiful in nutrient C. This nutrient is known for its potent antioxidant that shields the skin from the destructive impacts of free radicals. Vitamin C is likewise known to promote faster skin healing and it improves one's skin texture. Different supplements that will do wonders for your skin also includes nutrients E, K, and A, selenium, omega-3, zinc, and monounsaturated and polyunsaturated fats (good fats). Thus, whenever you make your menu plan, make a point to incorporate healthy servings of foods stuffed with these supplements.

4. TAKE BEAUTY SUPPLEMENTS

Eating your way to amazing skin is important; in any case, you should concede that it is hard to devour all the supplements your skin needs from the food you eat alone. Your skin is the biggest organ of our body, which is the reason it requires more nutrients and minerals to remain healthy. Your skin is constantly presented to various environmental variables that cause premature skin aging. Along these lines, aside from increasing your daily vegetable and fruit intake consumption, it tends to be useful to take supplements that benefit the skin. Popular supplements for skin are made up of multivitamins particularly ones with vitamin E and biotin, antioxidants like resveratrol and hydration specialists like hyaluronic acid and collagen.

Numerous analysts indicated that both oral and topical beauty supplements could help improve the quality and health of your skin. One investigation on the impacts of an anti-oxidant supplement on skin radiance of ladies uncovered positive effects. The women who experienced the test had at the end of the examination reduced skin defects, increased skin health, and additionally shining skin after they were given a continuous dosage of an anti-oxidant rich oral supplement. Application of ingredients like almond, green tea,chamomile and other organic sources can likewise give skin-caring advantages. Essential oils are packed with antibacterial and anti-inflammatory contents, and different properties that help forestall and treat skin issues.

5. CLEANSING BEFORE BED

A fundamental part of any skincare routine is cleansing. Since old times, individuals have been cleaning their skin to improve its health and appearance. While the techniques for cleansing have changed, the fundamental rule continues as before – your skin needs cleaning. You may not know about it, but your cosmetics are transporters of free radicals in nature. Regardless of whether you don't wear cosmetics, skin gathers residue and dirt for the day that sits on the skin alongside your sweat and sebum.

When you forget to clean your skin before going to bed, your skin is essentially "laying down with" free radicals. The exposure to free radicals damages the healthy collagen in our skin, bringing about fine lines and wrinkles.

Asides from exposing your skin to the damage, your facial pores can likewise get obstructed because of cosmetics and oils. At the point when this occurs, your skin gets defenseless to skin breakouts, enlarged pores, and other skin issues. Facial cleansing is significant in keeping up a healthy and flawless complexion. In this way, whenever you are enticed to sleep with your make-up on, consider the destructive outcomes and grab your facial cleanser or if nothing else rose water or a face cleansing wipe.

6. GET ENOUGH SLEEP

Getting enough sleep (for at least 7 hours) and not just sleeping ought to be a significant part of your skincare habits. Regardless of whether you have researched on this topic or not, the connection between good sleep and skin condition is self-evident and obvious. Try sleeping only a couple of hours every night, and you will before long feel and see positive changes in your complexion. The strong relationship between getting enough sleep and skin conditions was stressed considerably further by the aftereffects of an examination on regular sleep issues and dermatological conditions. The same exam uncovered that individuals who experience the ill effects of sleep disorders are increasingly powerless to encountering skin disorders like dermatitis, psoriasis, and skin aging.

Sleeping is significant for a healthy complexion since it is just during profound and long nights of sleep can your phones rest, and damaged cells get replaced. Interfering with this procedure implies your skin barely improves, bringing about apparent indications of aging skin. Allow your skin to remain youthful by getting your magnificence rest.

7. DEAL WITH YOUR STRESS

Psychological stress is one of the primary sources of numerous skin diseases, and it negatively influences your skin condition. At the point when you are stressed, your body enacts "emergency" physiological reactions to enable you to adapt. Unfortunately, prolonged enactment of these reactions can bring about skin aging, amongst others. An investigation on Dermatology Online Journal uncovered that psychological stress is straightforwardly connected to skin aging. Stress causes brokenness of the insusceptible system, damage to DNA, just as endocrine and resistant modulation – all of which add to skin aging.

Aside from skin maturing, your skin likewise turns out to be progressively helpless to microbial disease when you're continually stressed. One clinical examination demonstrated that stress upsets the antimicrobial capacity of the epidermis or the external layer of the skin. Given the interruption of the skin's guard framework, it gets inclined to disease. Keep all these negative impacts from occurring by incorporating stress management in your skincare routine. Do breathing activities, tune in to music, or attempt fragrant healing to soothe yourself from stress. Topical use of basic oils like sweet almond and chamomile can likewise help you right now.

8. USE A MOISTURIZER

A few people feel that applying a moisturizer is mostly for stylish purposes when truth be told, it is a crucial part of skincare. Our skin is the most exposed part of the body, and this exposure can prompt dryness and loss of dampness. Applying moisturizer is expected to restore the skin's lost moisture and essential oils, particularly in the wake of cleansing, conditioning, or moisturizing. A skin that is very moisturized is delicate, smooth, glowing, and more youthful-looking. A skin that is insufficient in the required moisture is dry, dull, and textured – at the end of the day, ugly.

If you are reluctant to incorporate moisturizing in your daily skincare routine since you live in a humid environment orhave oily skin note that dermatologists state you still should. Nonetheless, rather than using moisturizing items that are cream-based, decide on a lighter solution or serum with humectants like hyaluronic acid. For included security, use a moisturizer with sunscreen.

9. KEEP YOUR BODY MOVING

While exercise is all the more generally connected with losing weight, an ever-increasing number of people are finding how it promotes healthy and youthful-looking skin. If you question this reality, simply watch athletes or the individuals who have an active and exercise packed life; don't they look a lot more youthful and have better skin? Exercise helps in better blood flow. At the point when you walk, run, or dance, your body builds its bloodstream. At the point when this happens, the nutrients in the blood are better delivered to your skin cells, which means your skin turns out to be very much nourished. Also, the active blood flow helps in detoxifying your system bringing about a superior complexion.

If it is the case that you experience the ill effects of inflammatory skin infections like eczema and psoriasis, you should avoid potential risk when moving because the increase in your body temperature can intensify your condition. To maintain a strategic distance from uneasiness, make a point to practice in a relaxed environment like a well-ventilated exercise center or jogging at night instead of during the daytime. Abstain from swimming too since the chlorine in the water can aggravate a number of your symptoms.

10. USE SKIN PRODUCTS MADE FROM NATURAL INGREDIENTS

Your daily skincare routine will never be complete without skincare items. Contrary to what numerous people accept, everybody needs and uses such items, whether they know about it or not. When using skin items, be sure that they contain, for the most part, natural ingredients. Skincare items produced using botanical ingredients provide anti-inflammatory, anti-aging, and anti-bacterial advantages, and are even earth-friendly. Then again, items that contain, for the most part, human-made chemical compounds like parabens, sulfates, phthalates, and formaldehyde can trigger skin conditions and damage your skin. To guarantee that you might be using skincare items gotten from nature, make it a habit to check out the name. If you notice toxic chemical compounds in the ingredients list, avoid the item at all expense.

All the fundamental skincare tips mentioned above may show up too commonplace to even think about making an effect; however, they are supported up by science. If you figure you might be willing to undergo agonizing dermatological procedures just to get a more youthful-looking skin, why not attempt these simple things that can assist you with achieving similar outcomes?

CHAPTER THREE

Benefits Of Hand-Made Projects Or DIY

DIY (Do It Yourself) has gotten popular in recent years, with project instructions generally accessible on the internet along with an enormous range of educational programs on television. The cost of procuring an expert can be difficult to fit into a family budget and obtaining new abilities while settling on budget-accommodating choices can be appealing! From the beginning, you may have the feeling of being out of your usual scope of familiarity; in any case, the delight of viably finishing a project all alone can be a critical lift to your confidence. Instances of DIY projects may incorporate any kind of home improvement, for instance, painting, remodeling, tile and mosaic craftsmanship, furniture building, or surface articulations. Cooking and gardening – no longer necessities for perseverance in our modern world – are healthy, sustaining DIY family works out. If you are keen on innovation, shouldn't something be said about building a site? DIY potential outcomes are unending!

1. Benefits for your brain

In any case, you'll use your imagination to picture the final product of your new project. Imagine the ideal result; what are the means to enable you to get to that point? What abilities will you learn, and which assets will assist you with understanding the procedure? Solid arranging and hierarchical aptitudes will transform your project into a summary of materials and objectives for shopping and building. A little fluency in mathematics may be required – you can re-learn your 123s and increase your IQ moreover! Learning new abilities exercises your brain and securing extra knowledge will keep you pushing ahead into greater and more noteworthy DIY projects as your confidence increases. Assembling all that you learned in DIY projects and reusing it is assigned "combined learning," and it makes you increasingly intelligent.

2. Benefits for your body

While you are physically building a project, you can also improve and increase your strength, energy, and cardiovascular health. The action and activity will increase your strength, and your objectives for completing the project will help keep you engaged and invigorated as well. Gardening is a superb case of a decent DIY project. You will have the chance to create garden beds and structures, exercise yourself, and contemplate planting prerequisites and growing cycles. You will similarly be developing healthy nourishment to fuel your body and brain!

3. Benefits for your public activity

DIY projects are a magnificent strategy to meet new individuals with relative interests or aptitudes to share. Your projects and triumphs will be normal conversation openers, both on the web and face to face. On the off chance that you're hesitant, the ability to talk about your projects can assist you with venturing out of your social safe spot. You will learn a great deal by imparting encounters with other people, and it is a way to gain from the knowledge of others. Numerous skilled DIYers are liberal with sharing their aptitude! It is more than worth your chance to become a close acquaintance with similarly inclined individuals.

4. Benefits for your budget

With a DIY project, your work is free! The cost of materials is usually the only expense. At the same time, when you are new to DIY projects, you may commit material buying errors that could, in the end, be budget breakers; pick circumspectly and shop admirably. Contingent upon the size of your project, never cut corners by overlooking local building and zoning codes. Some home projects may require permits. It would moreover be gainful to come back to your home warranty to check whether your DIY project is for the most part successfully paid for. Visit your local building code office to ask questions regarding potential permit requirements for your project.

5. Benefits for your family

In case you have a busy or a hectic schedule or a big family, a significant DIY project can be problematic; think about a smaller project to start. A project restricted to one little space in your home or one that can be finished in a week will be less difficult to handle without getting tired. Counting the whole family in is a goal to consider too! On the off chance that you have small kids, attempt to consider the parts of the project they would appreciate adding to? Make a point to find errands that are basic, protected, and proper for your children.

CHAPTER FOUR

Hand Hygiene

Hand washing (or handwashing), otherwise called hand hygiene, is the demonstration of cleaning hands to expel dirt, earth, oil, and micro-organisms. Handwashing with soap reliably at specific "crucial points in time" during the day forestalls the spread of numerous illnesses, for instance, diarrhea and cholera, which are transmitted through the fecal-oral course. Individuals can likewise get contaminated with respiratory illnesses, for example, flu or the common cold, for instance, on the off chance that they don't wash their hands before touching their eyes, nose, or mouth (i.e., mucous membranes). The five crucial points in time during the day where washing hands with soap is important to include: after one uses the toilet, after cleaning a kid's bum or change dirty nappies, before touching a baby, before eating and when preparing food or touching raw meat, fish, or poultry. If water and soap are not accessible, hands can be cleaned with ash.

Clinical hand hygiene alludes to hygiene practices identified with clinical techniques. Hand washing before overseeing medicine or clinical consideration can forestall or limit the spread of illness. The principal clinical reason for washing hands is to purify the hands of germs (pathogens, infections, or different microorganisms and bacteria that can cause illness) and chemical compounds, which can cause infections or diseases. This is particularly significant for an individual who touches food or work in the clinical field, but it is also a significant practice for the entire population.

Hand washing has numerous health benefits, including the following:

- Minimizes the spread of flu;

- Prevents infectious cases of diarrhea;

- Decrease respiratory infections;

- Reduces infant death rate in home birth deliveries.

A recent report demonstrated that improved handwashing practices might prompt little improvements in the growth development in children under five years of age. In developing countries, child mortality rates identified with respiratory and diarrheal infections can be decreased by presenting simple behavioral changes, for example, handwashing with soap. This basic activity can lessen the rates of mortality from these illnesses by practically 50%. Interventions that promote handwashing can lessen diarrhea episodes by about a third, and this is equivalent to giving clean water in low-income areas. 48% of reductions in diarrhea episodes can be related to handwashing with soap.

Handwashing with soap is the absolute best and reasonable approach to prevent diarrhea and acute respiratory infections (ARI), they should be adopted as automatic behaviors carried out in homes, schools, and communities around the world. Pneumonia, a significant ARI, is the primary source of mortality among children under five years of age, ending the lives of 1.8 million kids every year. Diarrhea and pneumonia together account for nearly 3.5 million child mortality rates annually. According to UNICEF, turning handwashing with soap before eating and after using the toilet into an imbued habit can spare a larger number of lives than any single antibody or clinical intercession, cutting death from diarrhea by practically half and death from acute respiratory infections by one-quarter. Hand washing is typically associated with other sanitation mediations as a significant aspect of water, sanitation, and hygiene (WASH) programs. Hand washing additionally secures one against impetigo, which is transmitted through direct physical contact.

Soap and detergents

The removal of microorganisms from the skin is enhanced by the addition of soaps or detergents to water. The principal function of soaps and detergents is to increase solubility. Water alone is an inefficient skin cleanser since fats and proteins, which are types of natural dirt, are not properly broken down in the water. Soap is, be that as it may, helped by a sensible flow of water.

Soap

Soaps irrespective of their sizes and as a result of their reusable nature may hold germs procured from past uses. Few infections which have residue bacteria and germs on them as a result of contaminated soaps can be washed off with the foam one gets while lathering. The CDC, despite everything states, "liquid soap with hands-free controls for administering is preferable."

Antibacterial soap

Antibacterial soaps have been intensely elevated to a health-conscious public. Until now, no evidence of using prescribed antiseptics or disinfectants weakens anti-biotic resistant agents in nature. However, antibacterial soaps contain regular antibacterial agents, for example, triclosan, which has a broad rundown of safe strains of living beings. In this way, regardless of whether anti-infection safe strains aren't chosen for by antibacterial soaps, they probably won't be as compelling as they are advertised to be. Other than the surfactant and skin-securing agent, the modern formulations may contain acids (acerbic acids, ascorbic acids, lactic acids) as pH controller, antimicrobial dynamic benzoic acids and other skin conditioners (Aloe Vera, nutrients, menthol, plant extracts).

Water

Heated water that is comfortable for washing hands isn't sufficiently hot to remove bacteria. Microbes develop a lot quicker at the internal heat level of 37 % Fahrenheit. Be that as it may, warm, soapy water is more successful than cold, soapy water at expelling essential oils that hold dirt and microbes. Despite prevalent thinking, in any case, logical investigations have indicated that using warm water has no impact on diminishing the microbial burden on hands.

Cleaning Agents

A hand sanitizer or hand clean is a non-water-based hand hygiene agent. In the late 1990s and early piece of the 21st century, alcohol rub non-water-based hand hygiene agents (otherwise called alcohol-based hand rubs, germicide hand rubs, or hand sanitizers) started to pick up fame. Most depend on isopropyl alcohol or ethanol figured together with a thickening agent, for example, Carbomer (a polymer of acrylic acids) into a gel, or a humectant, for example, glycerin into a fluid, or froth for convenience and to diminish the drying impact of the alcohol. Including weakened hydrogen-peroxide increments further the antimicrobial movement.

Hand sanitizers containing at least 60 to 95% alcohol are efficient germ killers. Alcohol rub sanitizers eliminate bacteria, multi-drug resistant microbes (MRSA and VRE), tuberculosis, and some infections/viruses (counting HIV, herpes, RSV, rhinovirus, vaccinia, flu, and hepatitis) and fungus. Alcohol rub sanitizers containing 70% alcohol kill 99.97% (3.5 log reduction, like 35-decibel reduction) of the bacteria on hands 30 seconds after application and 99.99% to 99.999% (4 to 5 log reduction) of the bacteria on hands 1 minute after application. Hand sanitizers are best effective against bacteria and less potent against some other infections. Alcohol-based hand sanitizers are predominantly inefficient against norovirus or Norwalk type infections, the most widely recognized reason for infectious gastroenteritis.

HOMEMADE HAND SANITIZER

Enough hand alcohol rub must be used to thoroughly wet or rub two hands. The back and the front of both hands and between and the parts of all fingers are rubbed for around 30 seconds until the liquid, foam or gel is dry just as fingertips must be washed well, also focusing on them the two palms alternatively.

The US center for disease control and prevention prescribes hand washing over hand sanitizer rubs, especially when hands are dirty. The increasing use of these agents depends on their convenience and quick eliminating action against micro-organisms; be that as it may, they ought not to fill in as a substitution for legitimate hand washing except if soap and water are inaccessible. Frequent use of alcohol-based hand sanitizers can cause dry skin except if emollients, as well as skin moisturizers, are added to the recipe. The drying impact of alcohol can be diminished or killed by including glycerin as well as different emollients to the equation. In clinical trials, alcohol based hand sanitizers containing emollients caused considerably less skin irritation and dryness than antimicrobial detergents and soaps. Allergic contact urticaria syndrome,contact dermatitis,or hypersensitivity to alcohol or additives present in alcohol hand rubs once in a while happen. The lower tendencies to induce irritant contact dermatitis turned into a fascination as compared to soap and water hand washing.

Notwithstanding their viability, non-water agents do not cleanse the hands of organic material, however, they essentially disinfect them. It is therefore why hand sanitizers are not as powerful as soap and water at forestalling the spread of numerous pathogens since the pathogens despite everything stay on the hands. Alcohol free hand sanitizer efficacy is heavily dependent on the ingredients and formulations and verifiably has fundamentally failed to meet expectations of alcohol and alcohol rubs. All the more as of late, formulations that make use of benzalkonium chloride have been shown to have a tenacious and cumulative antimicrobial activity after application, in contrast to alcohol, which has been shown to reduce in efficacy after repeated use, likely because of various adverse skin responses.

Ash or mud

Numerous individuals in low-income communities can't afford the cost of soap and the use of ash or mud. Ash or mud might be more successful than water alone, however, might be less potent than soap. Evidence quality is poor. One concern is that if the dirt or ash is tainted with micro-organisms it might build the spread of sickness as opposed to diminishing it. Like soap, ash is likewise a disinfecting agent because, in addition to water, it frames a necessary arrangement. WHO prescribed ash or sand as an alternative to soap when soap isn't accessible.

Techniques

The right hand-washing technique recommended by the US Centers for Disease Control for prevention of transmission of sickness includes the following advances;

- Wet hands with cold or warm running water. Running water is recommended because standing basins might be contaminated, while the temperature of the water doesn't appear to make a difference.

- Lather hands by rubbing them with a lot of soap, including between fingers, the backs of hands, under nails.

- Soap removes germs from the skin, and studies show that individuals tend to wash their hands more altogether when soap is used as opposed to water alone.

- Scour for in any event 20 seconds. Scrubbing makes friction, which helps expel germs from skin, and scrubbing for more extended periods evacuates more germs.

- Rinse thoroughly under running water. Rinsing in a basin can re-contaminate hands.

- Dry your hands with a clean towel or allow to air dry. Wet and damp hands are all the more effectively re-contaminated.

The most commonly missed territories are the thumb, the wrist, the regions between the fingers, and under fingernails. Artificial nails and chipped nail clean may harbor microorganisms. Moisturizing lotion is often recommended to shield the hands from drying out; dry skin can prompt skin harm, which can increase the hazard for the transmission of infection.

Hand Sanitation and Hygiene

Hand sanitizer is a gel or a liquid generally used to diminish infectious agents on the hands. Formulations of the alcohol-based sort are desirable over handwashing with soap and water in many situations in the healthcare setting. It is generally progressively potent at killing microorganisms and preferred endured over soap and water. Hand washing should even now be completed if contamination can be seen or following the utilization of the restroom. The general use of non-alcohol-based versions has no recommendations. Outside the health care setting, hand washing is generally liked. They are likewise less powerful for smaller-scale organisms, and Clostridium difficile. They are accessible as liquids, gels, and foams. Alcohol-based versions regularly contain a mix of isopropyl alcohol, ethanol (ethyl alcohol), or n-propanol. Versions that include 60 to 95% alcohol are best. Care ought to be taken as they are combustible. Alcohol-based hand sanitizer neutralizes an assortment of microorganisms, however not spores. A few versions contain compounds, for example, glycerol, to prevent drying of the skin. Non-alcohol-based versions may contain benzalkonium chloride or triclosan.

CHAPTER FIVE

Home-Made Hand Sanitizer

Active Ingredients and Their Uses

Here's a portion of the lingo you've probably heard, seen, or read in advertising or on the names of some of the products you make use of.

ALPHA HYDROXY ACIDS (AHA'S)

These are organic product acids naturally obtained from fruit extracts. They slough off dead skin cells to reveal a younger and more youthful-looking skin. As we age, our skins renewal process slows down, and this helps to replace that process giving your skin a more youthful appearance.

- A – Aloe Vera

The gentle sap and gel of the Aloe Vera plant have been used for hundreds of years for its soothing properties. From calming rashes to treating acne, Aloe Vera uses countless solutions to your skincare needs. Aloe Vera gel is a popular natural skin care product that can be purchased pure. It is a fantastic remedy for sunburn, intensely moisturizing the skin and giving that genuinely necessary cooling sensation.

- B - Beeswax

If you experience the ill effects of skin complaints, for example, contact dermatitis, beeswax might be a particularly beneficial ingredient. When added to skin lotions, it goes about as a surfactant, creating a protective boundary on the outside of the skin, creating a film against irritants while as yet letting the skin relax. In the process, it will help to recuperate the skin with its anti-inflammatory, antibacterial, and anti-microbial properties.

- C - Coconut oil

Perhaps one of the most popular natural ingredients for skin since green tea, coconut oil, accompanies a plethora of recommendations. A brilliant moisturizer for the lips and skin, coconut oil effectively softens the skin when scoured on the body in its fibrous structure. It can likewise be combined with salts and sugars to make a regenerative exfoliator. Coconut oil is additionally a fantastic makeup remover – simply knead some into your face and then wipe off with a cotton pad absorbed warm water.

- D – Dandelion sap

Dandelion sap, also called dandelion milk, is growing in popularity for treating microbial and fungal infections. Its profoundly alkaline, germicidal, insecticidal and fungicidal properties settle on it an incredible choice for treating eczema and other skin conditions without the reactions of steroid creams. Be that as it may, make sure to keep away from contact with the eyes when using skincare products containing this ingredient.

- E - Eucalyptus

Eucalyptus is a much-underrated essential oil that is everything from antibacterial and anti-inflammatory to analgesic and insecticidal. In case you're looking to convert to a progressively natural lifestyle, eucalyptus oil would be a savvy choice to include into your medical aid unit, as it is brilliant for cleaning and healing cuts, minor wounds, rankles, wounds and insect chomps. In any case, this oil should consistently be blended in with a bearer oil, for example, grape seed oil before application. Check online for appropriate measurements for your purpose.

- F - Frankincense

The oil of the well-known resin frankincense has been utilized in beauty care products for a considerable length of time for its antiseptic and astringent properties. This makes it brilliant for preventing wounds from developing infections, yet it can likewise be used to protect against balding, to tone the skin and to lessen the appearance of wrinkles. It helps to promote the regeneration of cells, creating potent anti-aging characteristics when found in scientifically tried skin creams.

- G – Ginger

This spicy root is as useful for your skin as it is flavorful. It's a powerful anti-inflammatory and anti-oxidant highlights mean it tends to be utilized in skin products to include radiance, but at the same time is effective in treating fungal skin infections, and even for reducing cellulite. Added to a shower alongside different ingredients (see a recipe here), ginger can also help to treat varicose veins, as it supports the circulation in the legs.

- H - Hemp seed oil

The hemp seed oil has been used as a multi-purpose natural cure in eastern medicine for generations. Previously to some degree ignored because of the reputation of its controversial family member, this plant is now enjoying increased popularity. Hemp seed oil is often blended in with transporter oils or into creams as a moisturizer, as it has been proved to drastically diminish dryness, ease itching and even go about as an antioxidant and anti-inflammatory agent to calm the skin.

- I - Ice

One of the least demanding natural ingredients for the vast majority of us to obtain, all you need to get your hands on this substance is water and a freezer! It may appear as though a strange thing to want to do yet applying ice to the skin has many benefits. Warmth and ice treatments have gotten increasingly popular as a part of many spa breaks in Yorkshire and over the world, as it can wreck fat and dispose of spider veins. At home, applying ice to the face can lessen the inflammation under the eyes, shrink spots, and promote blood circulation for a youthful glow.

- J - Jojoba oil

Utilized by Native American communities for a considerable length of time to treat wounds, jojoba turned out to be internationally famous as a guaranteed organic skincare ingredient in the 1970s. Gotten from a bush that develops in the American southwest and Mexico, its oil is antibacterial, anti-inflammatory, and moisturizing, making it extraordinary for reducing acne without drying out the skin. It's additionally one of the best natural anti-aging ingredients out there, as it contains Vitamin E, which can help battle sun harm and lessen the appearance of scars and stamps on the skin.

- K - Kiwi seed oil

The oil of kiwi seeds isn't a commonly known skincare ingredient; however, it has a lot of benefits. Regardless of whether it be controlling sebum production to lessen the presence of pimples or firming the skin through the presence of collagen-inducing vitamin C, the kiwi seed oil is an unsung guardian angel of the natural skincare list.

- L - Lavender oil

A natural skincare superhero, lavender oil has a more significant number of employments than you could count. While it is essential to utilize this ingredient in the right quantities (else it can aggravate the skin), lavender is incredibly healing. Its powerful antiseptic and anti-inflammatory properties, while lavender is likewise a brilliant solution for acne, just as for reducing the itchiness of eczema. It is perhaps the best ingredient for healing burns and reducing the appearance scars.

- M - Marshmallow root

Marshmallows are one of the world's preferred sweet treats, yet its natural structure can likewise be a treat for your skin! Marshmallow roots, also called Althea, has healing, moisturizing and soothing properties, high in adhesive, which can cover the skin and prevent irritation. These make the ingredient brilliant for revitalizing the skin.

- N - Neroli oil

Originating in western India, eastern Africa, and the Himalayas, Neroli is gotten from orange blossoms. In ancient occasions, it was supposedly used to treat the plague. Today, nonetheless, it is applied topically to improve the skin is versatile, preventing the development of stretch imprints, along with reducing acne because of its anti-bacterial highlights.

- O - Oats

This may appear as though something you would be bound to have for breakfast than apply to your skin, yet oats have a vast number of employments for skin health. Those with sensitive skin could consider using cereal as a gentle exfoliator that will evacuate dead skin cells without irritating the skin's surface. Alternatively, it is brilliant for irritated, burned, or hypersensitive skin as a shower douse – simply place inside a muslin fabric and add to the shower.

- P – Patchouli

Extracted from a hairy bush local to Southeast Asia, patchouli is an individual from the mint family – not excessively, you would know it from its musky aroma. Other than being utilized in scents and cleansers, the essential oil can be applied topically with a bearer oil or in a cream to relieve irritation in infections and even in joint pain. It also contains astringent properties that make it useful for forestalling lines and wrinkled skin.

- Q - Quinoa

Quinoa has, as of late, become a health fever, with numerous individuals replacing pasta with this lighter alternative, which is stuffed with proteins and nutrients. Both eaten and applied topically; quinoa is additionally splendid for promoting unbroken skin. Because of its lysine content, it assists with mending harmed tissue, integrating elastin and collagen. One incredible approach to incorporate it into your skincare system is in an enemy of maturing face pack. This formula shows how a quinoa face pack can diminish indications of aging by fixing sun-burnt skin and smoothing the skin tone.

- R - Rose absolute

One of the most valuable essential oils on the planet, rose absolute, has a mind-blowing cluster of skin-mending properties. Its astringent properties make it incredible for treating wounds, as it makes the veins contract, easing back the bloodstream brought about by cuts and little bruises. It is likewise mitigating and calming, making it the ideal toner for dry, aroused, or bothersome skin. It also assists with conditioning and reinforces the skin for a youthful appearance.

- S – Sandalwood

Another sterile and mitigating fixing, sandalwood treats everything from creepy-crawly bites to boils. Notwithstanding, it is additionally a cicatrizant, implying that it can assist the skin with healing scars a lot faster. Sandalwood has, for quite some time, been utilized as a disinfectant, which, blended into the bathwater, can both forestall diseases and repulse creepy crawlies because of the oil's scent.

- T - Tea tree oil

A well-known solution for skin break out, tea tree oil is a ground-breaking clean that can help diminish abundance sebum creation to get out the skin. This Australian fixing is additionally hostile to contagious, making it powerful in expelling athlete's foot and other parasitic afflictions. Be that as it may, it can likewise alleviate dandruff and mitigate the tingling of bug bites. Tea tree oil can also treat minor wounds, support recuperating, and forestall contamination, so it's worth adding flexible oil to your typical medical aid unit!

- U - Ulmusdavidiana root extract

Honestly, this is a bit of a niche for some people, yet in case you're genuinely into attempting new things, Ulmusdavidiana root extract is unquestionably worth investigating. The bark of the root and stem of the Ulmusdavidiana japonica tree has been utilized in conventional Korean medication for a long time as a calming fixing.

The jury is still out on a portion of the healing properties of this root remove. Notwithstanding, numerous researchers trust it very well may be advantageous in the molding of the skin, and potentially as an enemy of wrinkle specialist to treat sun-initiated untimely maturing. If you do choose to search out this fixing, however, guarantee it is inside a trusted item that has been dermatologically tested!

- V - Violet leaf absolute

The concentrate of the violet leaf is maybe most regularly utilized in exquisite quality fragrances, yet it can also be applied to the skin for different outcomes. Perfect for delicate skin, this uncommon concentrate can mitigate and comfort irritated, rash-inclined skin, especially in the instances of dermatitis and dermatitis. Be that as it may, it is additionally gainful for oily skin, as its sterile components can tenderly refine the pores.

- W - Witch hazel

Witch hazel is another favorite for those experiencing spot-inclined skin. Gotten from the bark, twigs, and leaves of plants local to North America and a few pieces of Asia, the dynamic fixings are blended to create witch hazel water. Used topically, witch hazel is an incredible astringent, and cell reinforcement, usually decreasing skin break out, blisters, and bug bites. As an astringent, it assists with contracting the pores, diminishing the number of bacteria that can enter the pores and cause flaws.

- X - Xanthine

Xanthine probably won't sound like an especially 'regular' substance, yet don't stress – this is just a compound part of some sustaining common plants, for example, cacao beans and cola nuts. Plant extracts containing xanthine are known by researchers to forestall photograph harm from sun introduction when applied topically, lessening wrinkle arrangement. Search for creams containing xanthine in skin creams for everyday protection against untimely maturing.

- Y - Ylang-ylang

Facilitating various skin-recuperating properties, ylang-ylang essential oil is remarkable for its enemy of seborrhoeic characteristics. This implies it both diminishes irritation and regulates the sebum creation in skin infections. The substance is thought to help balance the hormones, decreasing skin break out and different grievances often incited by hormonal variances. It is likewise an extraordinary oil to knead into the scalp to keep the skin saturated and the hair looking healthy.

- Z - Zinc oxide

This mineral is an essential ingredient in sunscreen creams, as it is perhaps the most secure element for protecting the skin from UV beams. It has additionally been found by researchers that people with zinc lacks have moderate injury recuperating times, so zinc oxide is splendid for applying to wounds to enable the body to fix harmed skin cells.

EMOLLIENTS

Found in moisturizers, these ingredients help protect the skin by reinforcing the lower moisture barrier deep in, the lower epidermis of the skin. Natural emollients include Apricot Kernel Oil, Avocado Oil, Borage Seed Oil, Evening Primrose Oil, Grape Seed Oil, Hazel Nut Oil, Hemp Seed Oil, Kukui Oil, Macadamia Nut Oil, Mango Kernel Butter, Organic, Rose Hip Oil, Organic Sesame Seed Oil, Organic Shea Butter, Organic Sunflower Oil, Safflower Oil, Sesame Seed Oil, Shea Butter, Sunflower Oil, Sweet Almond Oil, Tea Tree Oil, Wheat Germ Oil.

Hand washing Versus Hand Sanitizer

Knowing when it's ideal for you to wash your hands, and when hand sanitizers can be useful, is vital to protecting yourself from infectious diseases as well as different illnesses, similar to the common cold and seasonal flu. While both fill a need, washing your hands with soap and water ought to consistently be a need, according to the CDC. Only use hand sanitizer if soap and water aren't accessible in a given situation. It's also essential to consistently wash your hands:

- after going to the washroom
- after blowing your nose, coughing, or sneezing
- before eating

- in the wake of touching surfaces that could be contaminated

The CDC records explicit instructions on the best method to wash your hands. This is what they recommend:

- Continuously utilize clean, running water. (It tends to be warm or cold.)

- Wet your hands first, then turn the water off, and lather your hands with soap.

- Rub your hands together with the soap for in any event 20 seconds. Make a point to scour the rear of your hands, between your fingers and under your nails.

- Turn the water on and rinse your hands. Utilize a clean towel or air dry.

Types Of Hand Sanitizers

Depending on the active ingredient utilized, hand sanitizers can be divided into one of two kinds: alcohol-based or alcohol-free. Alcohol-based items regularly contain between 60 and 95 percent alcohol, ordinarily in the type of ethanol, isopropanol, or n-propanol. At those concentrations, alcohol promptly denatures proteins, viably neutralizing certain kinds of microorganisms. Alcohol-free items are generally based on disinfectants, for example, benzalkonium chloride (BAC), or other antibiotic agents, for example, triclosan. The action of disinfectants and antimicrobial agents is both quick and persistent. Many hand sanitizers additionally contain emollients (e.g., glycerin) that mitigate the skin, thickening agents, and fragrance.

Effectiveness

The effectiveness of hand sanitizer depends on different variables, including the manner wherein the item is applied (e.g., quantity utilized, duration of introduction, frequency of utilization) and whether the particular infectious agents present on the person's hands are defenseless to the active ingredient in the sanitizer. In general, alcohol-based hand sanitizers, whenever rubbed altogether over finger and hand surfaces for a time of 30 seconds, followed by complete air-drying, can adequately diminish populations of microorganisms, fungi, and some enveloped infections (e.g., flu and other infections). Comparable impacts have been accounted for specific alcohol-free formulations, for example, SAB (surfactant, allantoin, and BAC) hand sanitizer. Most hand sanitizers, in any case, are generally ineffective against bacterial spores, non-enveloped infections (e.g., norovirus), and encysted parasites (e.g., Giardia). They likewise don't thoroughly cleanse or sanitize the skin when hands are noticeably filthy before application.

Regardless of the changeability ineffectiveness, hand sanitizers can help control the transmission of infectious ailments, particularly in settings where compliance with handwashing is poor. For instance, among children in elementary schools, the incorporation of either an alcohol-based or an alcohol-free hand sanitizer into study hall hand-hygiene programs has been related to reductions in absenteeism identified with an infectious illness. Moreover, in the working environment, the utilization of alcohol-based hand sanitizer has been associated with reductions in illness scenes and days off. In emergency clinics and health care clinics, increased access to alcohol-based hand sanitizer has been linked to overall improvements in hand hygiene.

The most common brands of alcohol hand rubs include Avant,Aniosgel, Sterillium, Desderman, and Allsept S. All emergency clinic hand rubs must conform to certain regulations like EN 12054 for hygienic treatment and surgical disinfection by hand-rubbing. Items with a case of "99.99% reduction" or 4-log reduction are ineffective in a medical clinic environment since the reduction must be more than "99.99%". The hand sanitizer dosing frameworks for medical clinics are designed to convey a deliberate amount of the item for staff. They are dosing sprays screwed onto a jug or are uncommonly designed dispensers with huge jugs. Dispensers for surgical hand disinfection are generally furnished with elbow-controlled mechanism or infrared sensors to stay away from any contact with the handle.

Surgical Hand Disinfection

Hands must be disinfected before any surgical method by hand washing with gentle soap and then hand-rubbing with a sanitizer. Surgical disinfection requires a more significant portion of the hand-rub and a longer rubbing time than is ordinarily utilized. It is typically done in two applications according to specific hand-rubbing techniques, EN1499 (hygienic hand wash), and EN 1500 (hygienic hand disinfection) to ensure that antiseptic is applied wherever on the outside of the hand.

Alcohol-free

Some hand sanitizer items use agents other than alcohol to execute microorganisms, for example, povidone-iodine, benzalkonium chloride, or triclosan. The World Health Organization (WHO) and the CDC recommend "persistent" antiseptics for hand sanitizers. Persistent movement is defined as the prolonged or extended antimicrobial action that prevents or inhibits the proliferation or endurance of microorganisms after the application of the item. This action might be demonstrated by sampling a site several minutes or hours after use and showing bacterial antimicrobial effectiveness when contrasted and a baseline level. This property additionally has been alluded to as "lingering action." Both substantive and nonsubstantive dynamic ingredients can show a persistent impact on the off chance that they substantially lower the number of microbes during the wash time frame.

Alcohol-free hand sanitizers might be taking effect right now while on the skin, however the solutions themselves can become contaminated because alcohol is an in-solution preservative, and without it, the alcohol-free solution itself is susceptible to contamination. Be that as it may, even alcohol-containing hand sanitizers can get contaminated if the alcohol content isn't adequately controlled or the sanitizer is contaminated with microorganisms during manufacture.

In June 2009, alcohol free Clarcon Antimicrobial Hand Sanitizer was pulled from the US advertise by the FDA, which found the product contained gross contamination of incredibly elevated levels of different bacteria, including those which can "cause opportunistic infections of the skin and underlying tissues and could bring about clinical or surgical attention just as permanent harm." The contamination of any hand sanitizer by bacteria during manufacture will bring about the disappointment of the effectiveness of that sanitizer and possible infection of the treatment site with the contaminating organisms.

Hand sanitizer, likewise called hand antiseptic, hand rub, or hand rub, agent applied to the hands to expel common pathogens (disease-causing organisms). Hand sanitizers normally come in froth, gel, or fluid form. Their utilization is recommended when soap and water are not accessible for hand washing or when rehashed handwashing bargains the natural skin obstruction (e.g., causing scaling or gaps to create in the skin). Although the effectiveness of hand sanitizer is variable, it is utilized as a basic means of infection control in a wide assortment of settings, from day-care centers and schools to medical clinics and health care clinics.

Hand sanitizer is a quick and handy way to deal with assistance forestall the spread of germs when cleanser and water are not available. Alcohol-based hand sanitizers can help keep you safe and reduce the spread of irresistible diseases. On the off chance that you are making some hard memories discovering hand sanitizer at your local stores and hand washing isn't available, you can figure out how to make your own. You just need two or three fixings, for instance, scouring alcohol, Aloe Vera gel, and an essential oil or lemon juice. Even though hand sanitizers can be a fruitful technique for disposing of germs, health specialists, despite everything, prescribe hand washing at whatever point possible to keep your hands liberated from affliction, causing infections and various germs.

Plans For Making Home-Made Hand Sanitizers

The Center for Disease Control prescribes 70% isopropyl or higher, or 60% ethanol or higher to make your own hand sanitizer. This implies, most alcohol in your in the alcohol bureau won't work. That non-developed whiskey that is 80 proof is just 40% alcohol. Vodka is moreover not sufficient at just 35-40%. Fortunately, on the off chance that you look in your medicine bureau and discover rubbing alcohol, this will work. Aloe Vera, or Aloe Vera gel, is furthermore required. If you have an Aloe Vera plant, the 100% aloe will encourage the consumption of the alcohol increasingly noticeable.

Directions

Mix 2/3 cup of your alcohol to 1/3 cup of Aloe Vera gel. I don't have a funnel at home, so I utilized a paper plate. The Aloe Vera is intended to soothe the dryness of the alcohol. In case you have a plant at home, stripping the leaves and squashing the gel is your most solid choice. You can incorporate essential oils, like tea tree, or lavender, or whichever fragrant you need, to cover the alcohol smell. Concerning forestalling the spread of irresistible diseases, nothing beats exemplary handwashing.

Nevertheless, if water and cleanser aren't open, your next best alternative, as per the Centers for Disease Control and Prevention (CDC) Trusted Source, is to use an alcohol-based hand sanitizer that contains at any rate 60 percent alcohol. Except if you have a save of locally obtained hand sanitizer, you'll likely gain some hard experiences finding any at a store or online at this point. In light of the speedy spread of irresistible diseases, most retailers can't remain mindful of the demand for hand sanitizer. The elevating news? Only three things are required to make your hand sanitizer at home.

A Note Of Warning

Hand sanitizer plans, including the one beneath, are expected for use by professionals with the vital capacity and assets for safe creation and legitimate usage. Possibly use specially crafted hand sanitizers in over the top circumstances when hand-washing isn't available for quite a while to come. Try not to use specially designed hand sanitizers on kids' skin as they may be logically inclined to utilize them improperly, prompting a progressively strong danger of injury.

What Ingredients Do You Need?

Making your hand sanitizer is not hard to do and just requires two or three fixings:

- isopropyl or scouring alcohol (99 percent alcohol volume)

- Aloe Vera gel

- an essential oil, for instance, tea tree oil or lavender oil, or you can use a lemon press.

The best approach to making an amazing, germ-busting hand sanitizer is to hold fast to a 2:1 extent of alcohol to Aloe Vera. This keeps the alcohol content around 60 percent. This is the base sum expected to execute most germs, as indicated by the CDC Trusted Source.

An Alternative Method Of Making An Home-Made Hand Sanitizer

Another technique for making hand sanitizers is a formula by Dr. Rishi Desai, chief medical officer of Osmosis, and a former plague knowledge administration officer in the division of viral diseases at the CDC. What you'll require:

- 3/4 cup of isopropyl or rubbing alcohol (99 percent)

- 1/4 cup of Aloe Vera gel (to help keep your hands smooth and to check the brutality of alcohol)

- 10 drops of essential oil, for instance, lavender oil, or you can use lemon squeeze

Directions:

ü Empty all ingredients into a bowl, ideally one with a pouring spout like a glass measuring container.

ü Blend in with a spoon and then beat with a rush to transform the sanitizer into a gel.

ü Empty the ingredients into an empty container for single-use and imprint it "hand sanitizer."

Another alternative strategy is the one given by Jagdish Khubchandani, Ph.D., accomplice instructor of health science at Ball State University, shared a relative condition. His hand sanitizer condition joins:

HOMEMADE HAND SANITIZER

- Two segments isopropyl alcohol or ethanol (91 percent to 99 percent alcohol)

- One part Aloe Vera

- A couple of drops of clove, eucalyptus, peppermint, or other essential oil.

On the off chance that you are making hand sanitizer at home, Khubchandani says to adhere to these tips:

- Make the hand sanitizer in a spotless space. Wipe down ledges with a debilitated color arrangement beforehand.

- Wash your hands altogether before making the hand sanitizer.

- To mix, use a spotless spoon and whisk. Wash these things altogether before utilizing them.

- Ensure the alcohol used for the hand sanitizer isn't debilitated.

- Blend all the ingredients completely until they are all around mixed.

- Try not to contact the mix with your hands until it is prepared for use.

For a greater clump of hand sanitizer, the World Health Organization (WHO)Trusted Source has a formula for a hand sanitizer that incorporates:

- isopropyl alcohol or ethanol

- hydrogen peroxide

- glycerol

- sterile distilled or gurgled cold water

Is it safe?

DIY hand sanitizer plans are wherever all through the web these days — yet would they say they are sheltered? These plans, including the ones above, are proposed for use by professionals with both the ability and resources to make uniquely designed hand sanitizers safely. A locally made hand sanitizer is possibly suggested in phenomenal circumstances when you can't wash your hands for the foreseeable future. Less than ideal ingredients or extents can incite:

- Absence of efficacy, implying that the sanitizer may not satisfactorily wipe out the risk to a couple or all living beings;

- Skin irritation, injury, or burns;

HOMEMADE HAND SANITIZER

- Introduction to dangerous chemical substances through inhalation.

Specially designed hand sanitizer is also not prescribed for use with kids. Youngsters might be increasingly inclined to appropriate hand sanitizer use, which could incite progressively genuine dangers of injury.

Step by Step Instructions To Use Hand Sanitizer

Two things to think about when utilizing hand sanitizer is that you have to rub it into your skin until your hands are dry. And, if your hands are oily or muddled, you should wash them first with cleanser and water. Thus, here are a couple of insights for utilizing hand sanitizer enough.

- Shower or apply the sanitizer to the palm of one hand.

- Thoroughly rub your hands together. Guarantee you spread the whole surface of your hands and all of your fingers.

- Continue rubbing for 30 to 60 seconds or until your hands are dry. It can take up to 60 seconds, and every so often more, for hand sanitizer to kill most germs.

What Germs Can Hand Sanitizer Kill?

According to the CDC Trusted Source, an alcohol-based hand sanitizer that meets the alcohol volume requirement can rapidly lessen the number of organisms on your hands. It can likewise help destroy a wide range of disease-causing agents or pathogens on your hands. Be that as it may, even the best alcohol-based hand sanitizers have limitations and don't eliminate a wide range of germs. According to the CDC, hand sanitizers won't dispose of potentially unsafe synthetics. It's also not successful at killing the following diseases:

- norovirus

- cryptosporidium (which causes cryptosporidiosis)

- clostridium difficile (otherwise called C. diff)

Likewise, a hand sanitizer may not function properly if your hands are messy or greasy. This may happen after working with food, doing yard work, gardening, or playing a sport. If your hands look dirty or slimy, go with hand washing instead of a hand sanitizer. To slow the spread of infectious diseases, we're advised to wash our hands more, ideally with soap and water, or failing that, with hand sanitizers, let's examine this popular one:

Combine in a bowl,

HOMEMADE HAND SANITIZER

- 2/3 cups rubbing alcohol (99.9% isopropyl alcohol)

- 1/3 cup Aloe Vera gel

- Mix. Decant into a soap or pump bottle

- Give it a decent shake once in a while.

Aloe Vera is a lotion that will prevent your skin from drying out. That is useful since breaks in the skin can expand the threat of bacterial infection. The principle dynamic ingredient right now isopropyl alcohol (isopropanol). Most business hand sanitizers contain either ethanol, isopropanol, n-propanol, or a mix of any two. Blends of 60%-80% alcohol by volume take out microorganisms, so the 66% alcohol concentration in the formula looks about right if unadulterated rubbing alcohol (otherwise called "cautious spirits") is utilized. A look at Amazon, be that as it may, shows that it is commonly sold as a pre-orchestrated working dilution among half and 70%, to be used legitimately on surfaces. Blending even the 70% solution with the Aloe Vera will make the last alcohol concentration too low to even consider being in any capacity significant.

Regardless of the way that it's hard to take a few to get back some composure of, unadulterated ethanol could be used in the formula rather than isopropanol.

Ethanol is the alcohol found in spirits, and other hand-made sanitizer that has increased some consideration utilizes vodka. Most vodka contains about 40% alcohol – not nearly enough for a successful hand sanitizer. In any case, Balkan 176, the most grounded vodka available in the UK, comes in at a stunning 88% ethanol. This could be used to make another 66% alcohol hand sanitizer with three sections vodka to one section Aloe Vera. At around £45 for 700ml, it would make a costly thing, yet since it was sold out on all the sites that we investigated, maybe there's a business open door for it.

An ongoing report indicated that both ethanol and isopropanol preparations made to the official World Health Organization (WHO) formulations inactivate the Sars and Mers infections, which are likewise infections. These formulations contain last concentrations of either 80% ethanol or 75% isopropanol, alongside 1.45% glycerol and 0.125% hydrogen peroxide. Everything in these formulations is blended in distilled water or essentially cold percolated water. The hydrogen peroxide is used to inactivate any contaminating microorganisms in the blend, yet it is certainly not a working ingredient in the sanitizer. The glycerol is a humectant, a substance to help hold moistness and can be supplanted with some other emollient or cream to help with skincare – including Aloe Vera.

Why Hand Sanitizers are Important

Everybody has had one of those days. It's pre-winter, and you're stuck at home enclosed by each blanket you possess, devouring bowl after bowl of soup, and lamenting every handshake you've given over the previous week. With cold and flu season here, it's essential to figure out how to guarantee you and your family are prepared – remembering putting in place hand sanitizers and soap for easy access, hand washing, and sterilizing strategies. We've put this manual for hand sterilizing together so you can understand one of the key weapons in your germ-fighting arsenal:

What Are the Benefits of Using Hand Sanitizer?

Alcohol-based hand sanitizers help to hinder the spread of germs and illness-causing bacteria, particularly in working environments like schools and workplaces:

- Stop the Spread of Germs: According to examinations, 1 in 5 people do not consistently wash their hands. And out of the individuals that do, 70% don't use soap. Providing hand sanitizer in critical territories (including restrooms and kitchens) makes it more probable that people will use it to kill harmful bacteria.

- Promote Good Hygiene and Health: A healthy place is a productive one. One research in the American Journal of Infection Control (AJIC) found that encouraging the use of hand sanitizers in schools diminished absenteeism by practically 20%!

- Reduce Waste: As an additional precaution, many people will utilize paper towels to open entryways when leaving restrooms or kitchens. Placing hand sanitizers near door entries and exits makes it simple for people to defend themselves from germs without needing to go through too much stress.

How Is Hand Sanitizer Most Effectively Used?

You must use hand sanitizer properly to ensure it carries out the role it's meant to do – dispose of germs before they spread:

- Don't Use Hand Sanitizer if Your Hands are Dirty: Hand sanitizers are not intended to clean your hands. They're intended to disinfect Residue like oil or soil will prevent hand sanitizers from penetrating down to your skin.

- Utilize the Right Amount: When it comes to hand sanitizer, less doesn't mean more. You need to apply enough to cover all aspects of your hands completely. Don't disregard the rear of them or your fingers!

- Focus on It Until Your Hands Are Dry: This way you can be certain that it's come into contact with all the most important surfaces.

When combined with other preventative measures (like proper handwashing and exhaustive touch-point cleaning), using hand sanitizer will help to keep you (and everyone in your building!) protected against this season's cold virus and different illnesses.

CHAPTER SIX

WHO Guidelines For Handwashing

The WHO guidelines and local guidelines do not contrast too severely since both contain the dynamic alcoholic ingredient and an emollient. The issue may be that the 66% alcohol concentration is towards the lower end of the effective range. Studies have shown that higher alcohol concentrations work better, and we know that the WHO 75% isopropanol or 80% ethanol formulations can kill and eliminate different viruses. The custom-made items may not be strong enough to inactivate the infection very as adequately as the WHO formulation. On the other hand, some business hand sanitizers contain as meager as 57% alcohol, so these natively constructed items would be superior to that.

In our opinion, if you want to make a custom made hand sanitizer, you ought to go with an adjusted version of the main formula, upping the rubbing alcohol to the WHO-recommended concentration: 75% of a cup of isopropanol and a fourth of a cup of Aloe Vera gel. You could even substitute glycerol for the Aloe Vera gel. It's less expensive, yet it won't smell as nice. Continuously follow the security instructions on whichever alcohol you utilize and recollect this is only for cleaning your hands. Don't wash in it and don't drink it!

To help countries and health-care offices to accomplish framework change and adopt alcohol-based hand-rubs as the best quality level for hand hygiene in health care, WHO has identified formulations for their local preparation. Strategic, economic, security, and social and strict elements have all been painstakingly considered by WHO before recommending such formulations for utilization around the world (see additionally Part I, Section 14). At present, alcohol-based hand rubs are the only known means for rapidly and adequately inactivating a full cluster of potentially unsafe microorganisms on hands. WHO recommends alcohol-based hand rubs based on the following variables:

- Evidence-based, intrinsic advantages of quick-acting and broad-spectrum microbicidal action with a minimal danger of generating resistance to antimicrobial agents;

- Suitability for use in asset constrained or remote regions with an absence of availability to sinks or different offices for hand hygiene (including clean water, towels, and so on.);

- Capacity to promote improved compliance with hand hygiene by making the process quicker and increasingly convenient;

- Economic benefit by reducing annual expenses for hand hygiene, representing approximately 1% of extra-costs generated by HCAI;

- Minimization of dangers from antagonistic events because of increased health-related to preferable acceptability and tolerance over different products.

For optimal compliance with hand hygiene, hand rubs ought to be promptly accessible, either through dispensers near the point of care or in little jugs for on-person carriage. Health-care settings currently using economically accessible hand rubs should continue to utilize them, provided that they fulfill recognized guidelines for microbicidal efficacy (ASTM or EN standards) and are very much accepted/endured by HCWs (see additionally Implementation Toolkit accessible at http://www.who.int/gpsc/en/). These products ought to be viewed as acceptable, even if their contents contrast from those of the WHO-recommended formulations portrayed below. WHO recommends the local production of the following formulations as an alternative when reasonable business products are either unavailable or excessively expensive.

The Volume Of Production, Containers

- 10-liter preparations: glass or plastic containers with screw-threaded stoppers can be utilized.

- 50-liter preparations: huge plastic (preferably polypropylene, translucent enough to see the fluid level) or stainless-steel tanks with an 80 to100 liter capacity ought to be utilized to allow for mixing without overflowing.

- The tanks ought to be aligned for the ethanol/isopropyl alcohol volumes and the final volumes of either 10 or 50 liters. It is ideal to stamp plastic tanks outwardly and stainless-steel ones on the inside.

Preparation

1. The alcohol for the chosen formulation is poured into the enormous container or tank to the graduated imprint.

2. H_2O_2 is included using the measuring cylinder.

3. Glycerol is included using a measuring cylinder. As the glycerol is thick and adheres to the dividers of the measuring cylinder, it very well may be rinsed with some sterile distilled or cold bubbled water to be included and then emptied into the jug/tank.

4. The jug/tank is then topped up to the corresponding characteristic of the volume (10-liter or 50-liter) to be prepared with the remainder of the distilled or cold, bubbled water.

5. The top of the screw cap is placed on the jug/tank following mixing to prevent evaporation.

6. The solution is blended by gently shaking the recipient where appropriate (little quantities), or by using a wooden, plastic, or metallic paddle. Electric blenders ought not to be utilized unless "EX" protected given the danger of explosion.

7. After mixing, the solution is quickly isolated into littler containers (for example, 1000, 500, or 100 ml plastic jugs). The pitchers ought to be kept in quarantine for 72 hours. This allows time for any spores present in the

alcohol or the new or re-utilized pitchers to be eliminated by H2O2.

Labeling Of The Containers

The containers ought to be marked by national guidelines. Marks ought to include the following:

- Name of institution

- Date of production and batch number

- Composition: ethanol or isopropanol, glycerol and hydrogen peroxide (% v/v can likewise be indicated) and the following statements:

- WHO-recommended hand-rub formulation

- For external utilize only

- Avoid contact with eyes

- Keep from the reach of children

- Use: Apply a palmful of alcohol-based hand-rub and spread all surfaces of the hands. Rub hands until dry. Combustible: keep away from fire and warmth.

Glycerol

Glycerol is added to the formulation as a humectant to expand the agreeableness of the item. Various humectants or emollients may be utilized for skincare, given that they are moderate, available locally, miscible (mixable) in water and alcohol, non-dangerous, and hypoallergenic. Glycerol has been picked since it is ensured and for the most part modest. Bringing down the level of glycerol may be considered to reduce the stickiness of the hand-rub also.

Various Additives Added To The Formulations

Notwithstanding, there is no distributed information on the compatibility and hindrance capability of such synthetic mixes when used in alcohol-based hand rubs to dishearten their maltreatment. It is essential to take note that such included materials may make the items poisonous and add to production costs. Additionally, the serious taste may be moved from hands to nourishment being handled by people utilizing hand rubs containing such agents. Thusly, compatibility, and sensibility, similarly as cost, must be intentionally considered before choosing the usage of such bittering agents. A colorant may be consolidated to separate the hand rub from various fluids as long in that capacity an additional substance is protected and good with the essential segments of the hand rubs. No information is available to review the sensibility of adding gelling agents to the WHO-prescribed fluid formulations, yet this might increment both production difficulties and costs and may bargain antimicrobial efficacy.

- The expansion of fragrances isn't prescribed as a result of the threat of ominously susceptible responses.

- All hand rub containers must be checked after national/international rules.

- To moreover lessen the peril of abuse and to regard social and exacting sensitivities, item containers may be stamped uniquely as "antimicrobial hand rubs".

- Utilization of legitimate water for the preparation of the formulations

- While sterile distilled water is preferred for making the formulations, percolated and cooled faucet water may similarly be used as long as it is liberated from perceptible particles.

Production and Storage

Assembling of the WHO-suggested hand-focus on formulations is conceivable focal pharmacies or dispensaries. At whatever point conceivable and as indicated by local approaches, governments should energize local production, bolster the quality assessment procedure, and keep production costs as low as could be permitted. Extraordinary prerequisites apply for the yield and accumulating of the formulations, similarly, concerning the capacity of the crude materials.

Since undiluted ethanol is astoundingly flammable and may touch off at temperatures as low as 10°C, production offices ought to straightforwardly debilitate it to the previously referenced concentration. The flashpoints of ethanol 80% (v/v) and isopropyl alcohol 75% (v/v) are 17.5°C and 19°C, respectively, (Rotter M, individual communication) and extraordinary consideration should be given to legitimate capacity in tropical climates. Production and capacity offices should be ideally, cooled or cold rooms. Open flares and smoking must be deliberately denied in production and capacity regions. Pharmacies and little degree production centers providing the WHO-prescribed hand rub formulations are instructed not to fabricate locally clumps concerning more than 50 liters in a steady progression. For health reasons, it is judicious to deliver humbler volumes and to adhere to local and national rules and guidelines. The production should not be attempted in focal pharmacies lacking particular cooling and ventilation. National security rules and local lawful necessities must be clung to for the capacity of ingredients and the last item.

Security Concerns

Agencies, for instance, the World Health Organization and the U.S. Centers for Disease Control and Prevention, increment the usage of alcohol-based hand sanitizers over sans alcohol items. Without a doubt, the usage of sans alcohol items has stayed obliged, halfway as a result of WHO's and CDC's consideration of alcohol-based items yet what's more taking into account worries about the health of synthetic mixtures used in sans alcohol items. Research has demonstrated that specific antimicrobial mixes, for instance, triclosan, for example, may meddle with the capacity of the endocrine framework. Environmental sullying from triclosan is another worry. Disinfectants and antimicrobials also can add to the improvement of antimicrobial obstruction. In 2014, mounting worries over triclosan drove specialists in the European Union (EU) to confine the substance's usage in various consumer items in the EU.

By comparison, worries over the usage of alcohol-based hand sanitizer have centered primarily on thing combustibility and ingestion, both unintentional (e.g., by small kids) and intentional (by people looking to manhandle alcohol). With proper capacity and methodologies that limit access to alcohol-containing sanitizer (e.g., giving hand sanitizer to people), the peril of fire or poisoning from incidental or intentional ingestion of alcohol-based hand sanitizers is viewed as low. Alcohol-based hand rubs are broadly used in the medical clinic environment as an option in contrast to antiseptic soaps. Hand-sanitizers on the clinic environment have two applications: hygienic hand rubbing and careful hand disinfection. Alcohol-based hand rubs give a superior skin tolerance when diverged from an antiseptic cleanser. Hand rubs moreover show to have logically ground-breaking microbiological properties when contrasted and antiseptic soaps.

Other ingredients utilized in over-the-counter hand-rubs are moreover utilized in emergency clinical hand-rubs: alcohols, for example, ethanol and isopropanol, on occasion joined with quaternary ammonium cations (quats, for instance, benzalkonium chloride. Quats are added at levels up to 200 segments for each million to build antimicrobial adequacy. Even though hypersensitivity to alcohol-based rubs is extraordinary, fragrances, additives, and quats can cause contact sensitivities. These various ingredients don't scatter like alcohol and gather, leaving a "clingy" development until they are cleared with cleanser and water.

CHAPTER SEVEN

Diseases And Infections That Can Be Averted By Proper Hand Hygiene

Hand washing: Reducing the Risk of Common Infections

Differences in the frequency and timing of hand-hygiene episodes may represent the more grounded decreases in rates of gastrointestinal ailments than rates of respiratory diseases. For instance, even with steady training messages that advocate hand hygiene legitimately after coughing or wheezing, such practices may not be as stable or as continuous as hand-hygiene practices immediately after defecation. Future hand-hygiene mediations should look to consolidate data on the frequency, span, and triggers for hand-hygiene scenes. Shockingly, the utilization of liquor-based hand sanitizers joined with hand-hygiene instruction was not firmly connected with decreased rates of gastrointestinal sicknesses or respiratory ailments. This was sudden given the fact that liquor-based sanitizers containing 60% to 80% weight per volume have been demonstrated to be viable against a scope of viruses and bacteria, including operators that cause looseness of the bowels or respiratory infections.

The utilization of benzalkonium chloride, a less frequently used hand sanitizer, showed a significant reduction in respiratory illnesses. In any case, this information was from just two investigations, 1 of which had a few structure imperfections. Discoveries from the clinical setting have bolstered the adequacy of liquor-based hand sanitizer for forestalling human services related infections, yet almost certainly, people living in the network have different hand-hygiene habits from those of staff in the social insurance setting. Even though population-based assessments are not accessible, an enormous observational study supported by the American Society for Microbiology has proposed that hand hygiene in the network is suboptimal.

Results from their investigation of 7836 people in 5 significant US urban communities indicated that solitary 67% of members washed their hands in the wake of using a general bathroom. Generally, more ladies (75%) than men (58%) washed their hands, proposing sex contrasts in practices. Unmistakably, predictable, and focused available hygiene ought to be supported in the network to expand the frequency of utilization.

Is it essential to wash your hands?

Basically, yes. Hand washing is the absolute best approach to forestall the spread of infections. You can spread "germs" (a general term for organisms like viruses and bacteria) calmly by contacting someone else. You can likewise get germs when you touch contaminated items or surfaces, and then you touch your face (mouth, eyes, and nose)."Great" handwashing methods incorporate using an adequate measure of cleanser, scouring the hands together to make contact, and flushing under running water. Wearing gloves is not a substitute for handwashing. There is extra data in OSH Answers about how the typical virus is transmitted by dirty and grimy hands. When would it be a good idea for me to wash my hands? Various circumstances where individuals can get "germs" include:

- When hands are unmistakably dirty.

- After using the washroom (which also includes dirty diapers).

- After cleaning out your nose or in the wake of sniffling in your grasp.

- Before and in the wake of eating, taking care of food, drinking, or smoking.

- After contacting raw meat, poultry, or fish.

- After taking care of trash or contact with contaminated surfaces, for example, trash receptacles, cleaning fabrics.

- Visiting or thinking about sick individuals.

- After cleaning someone else's nose or taking care of dirtied tissues.

- Before getting ready or taking drugs.

- After contact with blood or body liquids, for example, vomit or salivation.

- Before and in the wake of treating a cut or wound.

- Before inserting or removing contact lenses.

- Handling pets, creatures, or creature squander.

- After taking care of pet food or pet treats.

Keeping hands clean is one of the most significant advances we can take to abstain from becoming ill and spreading germs to other people. Numerous illnesses and conditions are spread by not washing hands with soap and clean, running water.

How Germs Get Onto Hands And Make Individuals Sick

Defecation (feces) from individuals or creatures is a significant wellspring of germs like Salmonella, E. coli O157, and norovirus that cause diarrhea, and it can spread some respiratory infections like adenovirus and hand-foot-mouth sickness. These sorts of germs can get onto hands after individuals use the toilet or change a diaper, and also in more subtle ways, as in the wake of taking care of raw meats that have undetectable measures of dirt on them. A single gram of human defecation—which is about the heaviness of a paper cut—can contain one trillion germs. Germs can likewise get onto hands if individuals touch any article that has germs on it since somebody coughed or sniffled on it or was moved by some other polluted item. At the point when these germs get onto hands and are not washed off, they can be passed from individual to individual and make individuals sick. Washing hands forestalls sicknesses and spread of infections to other people. Hand washing with soap removes germs from hands. This forestalls infections because:

- People frequently touch their eyes, nose, and mouth without acknowledging it. Germs can get into the body through the eyes, nose, and mouth and make us sick.

- Germs from unwashed hands can get into foods and beverages while individuals get ready or devour them. Bacteria can increase in certain kinds of foods or drinks, under specific conditions, and make individuals sick.

- Germs from unwashed hands can be moved to different articles, similar to handrails, tabletops, or toys, and afterward moved to someone else's hands.

- Removing germs through handwashing consequently forestalls loose bowels and respiratory infections and may even assistance prevent skin and eye infections.

- Showing individuals hand washing causes them, and their networks remain solid. Hand washing instruction in the system:

- Reduces the number of individuals who become ill with diarrhea by 23-40%;

- Reduces diarrheal ailment in individuals with debilitated safe frameworks by 58%;

- Reduces respiratory ailments, similar to colds, in everybody by 16-21%;

- Reduces non-attendance because of gastrointestinal sickness in schoolchildren by 29-57%;

- About 1.8 million children younger than 5 die every year from diarrheal illnesses and pneumonia, the best two enemies of little children around the world.

- Handwashing with soap could prevent around 1 out of every 3 children to become ill with diarrhea and just about 1 out of 5 children with respiratory infections like pneumonia.

- Although people around the globe clean their hands with water, not many use cleansers to wash their hands. Washing hands with soap expel more significant germs.

- Hand washing training and access to soap in schools can help improve participation.

- Proper handwashing may help improve kid advancement in specific settings.

- Estimated worldwide rates of handwashing after using the toilet is just 19%.

Hand washing helps fight the rise in antibiotic resistance

Preventing sickness decreases the number of antibiotics individuals use and the probability that antibiotic resistance will create. Handwashing can prevent about 30% of diarrhea-related illnesses and about 20% of respiratory infections (e.g., colds). Antibiotics regularly are recommended unnecessarily for these medical problems. Reducing the number of these infections by washing hands frequently prevents the abuse of antibiotics—the single most significant factor prompting antibiotic resistance around the globe. Hand washing can also keep individuals from becoming ill with germs that are already resistant to antibiotics, and that can be hard to treat. To achieve a complete and perfect result after the washing of your hands, follow these procedures;

- Remove any rings or other adornments.

- Use water and wet your hands altogether.

- Use cleanser (1-3 mL) and foam well indeed.

- Lather with soap for at least 15 seconds , ensure you wash between your fingers, front and backs of your hands,under your fingernails,

- wrists, and lower arms.

- Rinse altogether under spotless, running water. Utilize a scouring movement.

- Dry your hands with a paper towel or clean towel or utilize an air dryer.

- Turn off the taps/ faucets with a paper towel (so you don't re-sully your hands).

- Protect your hands from touching dirty surfaces as you leave the washroom. For instance, use a different paper towel to open the entryway.

Different tips include:

- Cover cuts with gauzes and wear gloves for added insurance (cuts are truly helpless against infections).

- Artificial nails and chipped nail polish have been associated with an increase in the number of microbes on the fingernails. Make sure to clean the nails appropriately.

- Keep your hands from your eyes, nose, or mouth.

- Assume that contact with any human bodily fluids is inevitable.

- Liquid cleanser in dispensable containers is ideal. If using reusable holders, they ought to be washed and dried before refilling. If using a bar of soap, make sure to set it on a rack that allows water to drain or use little bars that can be changed constantly.

- If dry skin happens, utilize a moisturizing cream.

Shouldn't something be said about antibacterial cleansers or hand sanitizers?

While the facts confirm that ordinary cleanser and water does not kill microorganisms (they make a tricky surface that permits the life forms to "slide off"), antibacterial cleansers are commonly viewed as pointless for most purposes. The exemption might be in a medical clinic where extraordinary circumstances are available (e.g., before intrusive strategies, when thinking about seriously immuno-traded off patients, basic consideration regions, escalated care nurseries, and so on.). Antibacterial specialists ought to be picked deliberately based on their dynamic fixings and qualities, and when diligent antibacterial or antimicrobial action on the hands is wanted.

When there is no cleanser or water accessible, one option is to utilize hand sanitizers, or waterless hand scours. A portion of these items is made of ethyl alcohol blended in with emollients (skin conditioners) and different operators. They are frequently accessible as a gel, or on wipes or towelettes. Alcohol-based hand sanitizers ought to contain in any event 60% alcohol. Sanitizers don't dispense with a wide range of germs and probably won't expel a few synthetic compounds. Hand sanitizers may have scents that might be aggravating to specific people.

- Apply the proposed sum to the palm of one hand based on the producer's suggestion.

- Rub hands together.

- Spread and rub the item over your hands and fingers until your hands are dry.

- Use enough to cover the entirety of your hands and fingers.

Alcohol-based hand sanitizers are the favored strategy for medicinal services suppliers when the hands are not noticeably dirty. The sanitizers can likewise be used by paramedics, home consideration chaperons, or other portable laborers where handwashing offices are not accessible. In any case, these specialists are not compelling when the hands are vigorously sullied with earth, blood, or other natural materials. Hand-washing with cleanser and water is suggested when hands are unmistakably filthy.

CONCLUSION

To conclude, these are some very important hygiene facts that should be used and acted upon.

Hygiene Facts

- It is assessed that washing hands with cleanser and water could decrease diarrheal related diseases by half.

- Researchers in London have worked out that if everybody routinely washed their hands, a million deaths every year would be prevented.

- A considerable number of foodborne disease outbreaks are spread by dirty hands. Fitting handwashing practices can diminish the danger of foodborne disease and other infections.

- Handwashing can reduce the risk of respiratory infections by 16%.

- The use of an alcohol gel hand sanitizer in the class gave a general decrease in absenteeism because the infection was reduced by 19.8 in

16 elementary schools and among 6,000 students.